Study of Suicide : Causes and Influencing Factors

Dr Charles W. Pilgrim
Robert N. Reeves
Allan McLane Hamilton
Pr Edwin Grant Dexter

Study of Suicide
Causes and Influencing Factors

LM Publishers

A Study of Suicide[1]

As the love of life is generally acknowledged to be the strongest instinct of the human mind, it is but natural that the subject of voluntary death should have attracted, at all times, a great amount of attention from moralists and sociologists.

Some of the noblest men and women of ancient times advocated and practiced self-destruction, and the frequency of the act in our own day demonstrates that the fear of death is by no means general. Prof. Mayer, of Paris, in a lecture on this subject, declared that every one of his hearers had, at some time, thought favorably of committing the deed. He challenged contradiction, but no one responded.

This longing for "restful death," which comes to nearly all of us sooner or later, can usually be resisted; but often the desire is so great that the will is not strong enough to overcome it, and another name is added to the

---

[1] By Dr Charles W. Pilgrim

long list of suicides which statistics show us is increasing with terrible rapidity.

Very exhaustive statistics in regard to this subject have been compiled by Profs. Bertillion and Morselli, and they both arrive at about the same conclusions. Taking each million of inhabitants, the following results were obtained: In Austria the number was increased between 1860 and 1878 by from 70 to 122 annually; in Prussia, between 1820 and 1878, by from 71 to 133; in the smaller German states, between 1835 and 1878, by from 117 to 289; in France, between 1827 and 1877, by from 52 to 149, the greater proportion being in the larger cities. Peasants rarely commit suicide, statistics showing that in Belgium, where laborers can generally find employment, the increase between 1831 and 1876 was only from 39 to 68. In Sweden and Norway about the same result was obtained, viz., an increase from 39 to 80 per year during the same period. Italy, Spain, and Ireland show the lowest number, the increase between 1864 and 1878 being only from 28 to 35 in the former, while in Spain and Ireland it was still less, the latter showing an increase of but from 14 to 18 per year during the same period. This result is probably due to a great extent to the influence of the Catholic priesthood, for it is the Roman Church, above all others, that has firmly "fixed its canon against self-slaughter."

On account of the more settled social condition of England the statistics of that country do not show the same alarming increase as those of France, Germany, and Austria, but the regularity of the number for each five years, from 1855 to 1875—viz., from 1855 to 1860, 65; from 1860 to 1865, 66; from 1865 to 1870, 67; and from 1870 to 1875, 66— supports in a remarkable degree the statement made by Buckle that, "when the social conditions do not undergo any marked change, we find year by year the same proportion of persons putting an end to their existence, so that we are able to predict, within a very small limit of error, the number of voluntary deaths for each ensuing period."

Both Profs, Bertillion and Morselli express some doubt as to the reliability of their statistics showing an increase in the United States on account of its rapidly increasing population; but anyone who will pay attention to the subject will be convinced, I am sure, that a marked increase is annually taking place; and there are many reasons why it should be so. Our country is young, social changes are rapid, and the struggle for wealth is severe. In brief, we are living in what is justly called a "fast age." The modern youth "consumes in an hour, by useless brilliancy, the oil of the lamp which should burn throughout the night," and soon finds that the infirmities of age have supplanted the vigor of youth; the business man who to-day is at the very height of prosperity, by some rash speculation becomes a bankrupt to-morrow; the professional man, who is ambitious of distinction, does not rest when the sun goes down, but prolongs his work far into the quiet hours of night. In fact, almost everyone is madly pursuing either pleasure, wealth, or fame, and, under such circumstances, is it a wonder that often an overpowering sense of *ennui* and disgust of life occurs, or that the delicate structure of the brain breaks down, impelling the unfortunate victim to seek rest in the suicide's dishonored grave?

Besides dissipation, reverses of fortune and overwork, love, jealousy, and remorse play an important part in the etiology of self-destruction. Marc Antony fell upon his sword and killed himself because he believed that Cleopatra had played him false; and she, overcome by remorse and grief, placed the asp to her breast that it might "the knot intrinsicate of life untie," and thus unite her in the grave with him whose absence filled her life with woe; and the same motives which, thirty years before the birth of Christ, made Antony and Egypt's queen "a-weary of the sun," rule just as powerfully to-day in modern hearts.

Such, causes, though occurring everywhere, are, of course, more frequent in large cities like Paris, London, and New York, the former probably taking precedence, it being no uncommon sight to see upon the marble slabs of the Morgue three or four dead bodies which have been recovered from the Seine. When the history of such cases can be learned, they show, in the majority of instances, the absence of domestic ties, coupled either with misguided love and jealousy or dissipation and remorse. Indeed, so far as men are concerned, we must consider marriage, with its accompanying influences of home and children, a most important prophylactic. In regard to women, however, this statement does not hold good, for with them suicide is more frequent among the married than the single, the proportion being 10 to about 9 or 9*4. This may be explained to some extent by the mental disturbances produced by pregnancy and child-birth, but the strongest reason undoubtedly is that a girl's youthful dreams of happiness are often shattered by the realities of married life.

One of the most interesting tables in this connection is that compiled by Bertillion, and first published in the "*Revue Scientifique*" for 1879. He found that among a million of inhabitants, taken from all classes, the following numbers committed suicide, viz.:

Married men with children	205	Married women with children	45
Married men without children	470	Married women without children	158
Widowers with children	526	Widows with children	104
Widowers without children	1,004	Widows without children	238

We here learn the interesting facts that, when marriage is childless, the number of suicides is doubled in men and trebled in women; and also that maternal love diminishes the number of suicides among widows with children by one third over those of childless unions.

This table also shows that males exceed females in the frequency of the act in the proportion of four to one. While this is true of suicides in general, it certainly is not the case in those who are insane. My experience leads me to believe that suicidal tendencies in the insane are quite as frequent among women as among men, and I am sure that the former frequently show the more determination and persistence. In the outside world men lead more exciting lives and are subject to greater mental strain than women, and it is therefore natural that they should more frequently resort to suicide. Another probable reason for the comparative infrequency of suicide among women is that they are better endowed with religious fervor and possess a larger share of hope. In India and Japan only does this rule fail to hold good, and there the number of suicides among women is twice as great as among men. This fact bears striking witness to the hardships of woman's lot in countries removed from the influences of civilization.

Statistics show that the months in which the fewest suicides occur are October and November, while the greatest number occur in April, May, and June. July and September also have a goodly share, the latter possessing a peculiar fascination for women. This refutes the old idea that suicides occur most frequently in damp and gloomy weather, for the months just mentioned as being the most prolific are certainly those in which the skies look brightest and the earth is fairest. Another remarkable fact in this connection is that the progressive increase and decrease in the number of suicides coincide with the lengthening and the shortening of the days, and, as M. Guerry has shown, not only the seasons of the year, but the days of the month and of the week, and even the hours of the day exert an influence, the constancy of which cannot be mistaken. As a result of his elaborate research he found that the greatest number of suicides among men occurred during the first ten days of the month, and from Monday to Thursday of the week. This is accounted for by remembering that the majority of workingmen receive their wages either on the first of the month or the last of the week, and that "pay-day" is often followed by dissipation, debauchery, and remorse. Oettingen completed this interesting observation by showing that the larger number of suicides among women take place during the last half of the week, when they are most apt to feel the effects of man's prodigality and wrong-doing. In regard to the hours of the day, we know, from Brierre de Boismont's examination of 1,993 cases of suicide in Paris, that the maximum number occurred between 6 A. M. and noon, and thereafter regularly declined, reaching the minimum at the hour before sunrise.

It is also an established fact that the more rugged natures of men impel them to seek coarser means of self-destruction, such as the revolver, the razor, and the rope, the latter being most frequently used by those in whom the vigor of manhood is lost. Women, on the contrary, seldom resort to measures which they think will disfigure them, and therefore most frequently seek death by poisoning, asphyxia, or drowning. This, of course, only refers to cases in which the suicide has opportunity to adopt the method preferred. In hospitals for the insane almost all suicides, both male and female, and of whatever age, are accomplished by suspension, that being generally the most available method.

Epidemics of suicide frequently occur, and he who introduces any unusual method is sure of having numerous followers. In 1793 an epidemic occurred in Versailles, and the population was decreased within a single year by 1,300 self-sought deaths. In the Hôtel des Invalides an inmate hung himself upon a certain cross-bar, and within a fortnight five more did the same thing, although there had not been a single case of suicide in the establishment for two years before, and the threatened epidemic was only averted by the removal of the fatal bar.

Lord Bacon, in his "Essay on Death," says that, "after Otho, the emperor, had slain himself, pity (which is the tenderest of affections) provoked many to die out of mere compassion to their sovereign." Plutarch tells us that the women of the ancient city of Miletus, becoming melancholy over the absence of their husbands and lovers, resolved to hang themselves, and vied with each other in the alacrity with which they did the deed. Various other epidemics have occurred in more recent times—viz., at Rouen, in 1806; at Stuttgart, in 1811, etc.

What might almost be called an epidemic prevailed in the New York State Lunatic Asylum in July, 1850. According to the report for that year, there were at one time twenty-eight persons in the institution bent upon destroying themselves. There were admitted during that month forty-four patients, nineteen of whom were suicidal. The first successful attempt occurred on the 12th, and on the following day two more, who had been in the asylum for a long time and had never shown suicidal tendencies, attempted strangulation, and were so persistent that they were only prevented from carrying out their designs by mechanical restraint. On the 17th, 20th, and 22d other attempts were made by various patients, and before the end of the month, at which time it subsided, there had been fourteen distinct attempts by eight persons, while several others, in whom the propensity was strong, required constant watching to prevent them from accomplishing their object.

These epidemics are, to a great extent, the result of the principle of imitation, and it may be said that suicide is almost as much the subject of fashion as is dress or household decoration, and that each particular method reigns for a time and then gives way to some newer means. For instance, a man destroys himself by plunging from the heights of a tower. The newspapers graphically record the fact, and straightway a dozen more do the same thing, and the practice is only stopped when someone who is tired of life sends a bullet through his brain. This method is then adopted until another takes a dose of carbolic acid, when that in turn becomes the prevailing means.

Another proof that suicide is often due to the faculty of imitation is the fact that many cases are recorded of children committing the deed, without apparent cause, after having heard of a case in which their interest was aroused.

Among the most remarkable attempts at suicide upon record is that of a man in Fressonville, in Picardy, as related by Dr.

Winslow, who was actuated by a desire to ring his own death knell. To accomplish this object he hanged himself to the clapper of the church-bell. But, fortunately, he chose an hour at which it was not customary for the bell to ring, and attention was attracted in time to save his life. Another very deliberate attempt, probably the most extraordinary ever known, was that made by an Italian shoemaker, named Matthew Lovat. This case was originally reported by Dr. Bergierre, afterward enlarged upon by Dr. Winslow in his "Anatomy of Suicide," and has since been frequently quoted by various writers. The history of the case in brief is that the man determined to imitate as nearly as possible the crucifixion of our Saviour, and therefore deliberately set about making a cross, and providing himself with all the adjuncts of that scene. "He perceived that it would be difficult to nail himself firmly to the cross, and therefore made a net which he fastened over it, securing it at the bottom of the upright beam and at the ends of the two arms. The whole apparatus was tied by two ropes, one from the net and the other from the place where the beams intersected one another. These ropes were fastened to the bar above the window, and were just sufficiently long to allow the cross to lie horizontally upon the floor of the apartment. Having finished these preparations, he next put on his crown of thorns, some of which entered his forehead; then, having stripped himself naked, he girded his loins with a white handkerchief. He then introduced himself into the net, and, seating himself on the cross, drove a nail through the palm of his right hand by striking its head upon the floor until the point appeared on the other side. He now placed his feet upon a bracket he had prepared for them, and with a mallet drove a nail completely through them both, fastening them to the wood. He next tied himself to the cross by a piece of cord around his waist, and wounded himself in the side with a knife which he used in his trade. The wound was inflicted two inches below the hypochondrium, toward the internal angle of the abdominal cavity, but did not injure any of the parts which the cavity contains. Several scratches were observed upon his breast which appear to have been done by the knife in probing for a place which should present no obstruction. The knife, according to Lovat, represented the spear of the passion. All this he accomplished in the interior of his apartment, but it was necessary to show himself in public. To accomplish this he had placed the foot of the cross upon the window-sill, which was very low, and by pressing his fingers against the floor he gradually drew himself forward until, the foot of the cross overbalancing the head, the whole machine tilted out of the window and hung by the ropes which were fastened to the beam. He then, by way of finishing, nailed his right hand to the arm of the cross, but could not succeed in fixing the left, although the nail by which it was to have been fixed was driven through it, and half of it came out on the other side. This happened at eight o'clock in the morning. Some persons by whom he was perceived ran up-stairs, disengaged him from the cross, and put him to bed. By medical care his wounds ultimately healed, but he was ever afterward morose and singular."

A person bent upon suicide will sometimes await a favorable opportunity for months, or overcome apparently insurmountable difficulties by the exercise of ingenuity which, if it were devoted to the accomplishment of a better object, would be worthy of the highest commendation. Dr. Wynter cites the case of a man who was placed under medical observation because he had attempted to commit suicide. He was watched with the greatest care; during nine months all means—so far as his attendants knew—by which he could injure himself were removed. But one morning he was discovered hanging by his neck from the bedstead, quite dead. How he became possessed of the cord was an enigma which was afterward solved by the discovery that he had carefully preserved every piece of string from the parcels that had been sent to him from time to time. With them he had twisted a rope sufficiently strong to accomplish his purpose. The newspapers a few months ago reported the case of a man named Frederick Helbig, of Zanesville, Ohio, who also showed considerable inventive talent. He was blind and disconsolate, and therefore resolved to die, but as none of the common methods were suited to his purpose he made his way to the cellar, broke off a piece of the gas-pipe, and then covering the end of the pipe and his head with a heavy quilt, quietly suffocated himself with the gas.

Another extraordinary case is that of a man who was quite recently admitted to the Buffalo Insane Asylum. He had attempted suicide the day before while in the station-house, and, owing to his dangerous tendencies, he was placed under the care of a special night-watch, who sat outside his door. For three nights all went well, but on the fourth he jumped from the head of his bed for the transom over his window, the only exposed glass in the room, crashing through the panes and seizing the bars on the outside. Before the attendant could prevent it he had, with a bit of glass, cut into his throat, severing the thyroid cartilage. The patient was in a frenzied condition, and it required the efforts of five attendants to keep him from tearing open the wound. The cartilage was united and the wound sewed and dressed. Foiled in his attempts to tear open the wound, he fixed his lips and jaws tightly and exhaled forcibly. He succeeded literally in blowing himself up, for the air found its way through the slit in the cartilage into the tissues about the wound, and in a few seconds the emphysema extended as low as the clavicles and so high that his features lost all expression. He refused food and resisted nutritive enemas and shortly died of exhaustion.

The question, "Is suicide an evidence of insanity?" is one which has given rise to much discussion. In olden times it seems always to have been considered a crime, and very severe laws were enacted against it. The Hebrews did not bury the bodies of suicides until after sunset, thus treating them as they did executed criminals. The Armenians cursed and burned the house in which the suicide had lived. At Thebes their bodies were burned and no funeral rites allowed; while the Greeks, on the contrary, among whom it was the custom to burn the bodies of those who died a natural death, buried suicides immediately, as they thought it a wrong to contaminate fire, which they deemed a holy element, by burning in it the bodies of those who had been guilty of self-slaughter. In England it was formerly attended by some of the consequences of felony, hence the term *felo de se*. All of the personal property which the party had at the time of committing the deed, even including debts to him, was forfeited to the crown, and his remains were interred, without the rites of Christian burial, in the public highway, with a stake driven through the body. In fact, everywhere was the act proscribed and considered a crime, until the present century, when it began to be regarded by many writers as a positive proof of insanity. Esquirol says, "I believe that I have proved that all suicides are mentally diseased"; and Dr. Winslow, one of the greatest authorities on this subject, supports Dr. Rowley's assertion that "suicide should ever be considered an act of insanity." On the other hand, Blandford, Griesinger, Bucknill, Tuke, Gray, and nearly all modern authorities think that suicide is often committed by people in whom no disease of the brain exists. Indeed, Dr. Gray went much further, and in one of his lectures said, "Suicide, though always an unnatural act, is, in the large proportion if not in the majority of cases, committed by persons who are entirely sane." Whether it is or is not the act of insanity can only be determined by a careful inquiry, as there are many cases to support either side of the argument, and each one must be a "law unto itself." For instance to be insane enough to commit suicide does not imply that a man must be a raving lunatic, "cutting strange antics before high Heaven," which make his madness apparent to the most unpracticed observer. Indeed, in many instances the attempt at suicide is the first prominent symptom of insanity, and frequently the intensity of the suicidal tendency subsides with the progress of the disease. All who know anything about the insane will admit that lunatics very frequently possess extraordinary cunning in concealing their lunacy, and that the malady, in many cases, is successfully hidden from friends and acquaintances until some remarkable departure from the ordinary ways of life brings it to light. A case in point is that of Hood Alston, who committed suicide in New Orleans in the early part of 1879, after writing a full explanation of why he wished to die. He had been an able writer for the newspapers in many of the large cities, his habits had been those of a gentleman, and his death, in the absence of the letter which he left, would have been inexplicable. He was in the Interior Department at Washington, and was afterward appointed the secretary of a mining company in California. He was married and had every requisite for domestic happiness. "Last November," he wrote, "I became possessed of an impulse to kill my friends. I could hardly resist an opportunity. The desire would be but for a moment and then pass away. An infant was born to us two months ago. I loved it, was proud of it. When it first looked upon me the desire seized me to prey upon its young life. My friends were ignorant of my mental condition. I imparted it to no one, not even to my darling wife. I die that others may live." Dr. Winslow relates a singular case of a man who was heard to exclaim: Do, for God's sake, get me confined, for if I am at liberty I shall destroy myself and wife; I shall do it unless all means of destruction are removed, and therefore do have me put under restraint. Something above tells me I shall do it, and I shall." Mr. Chevalier also tells us of a young lady of delicate constitution, although she had never given any symptoms of mental derangement, who suddenly started up from the tea-table and rushed to the window, out of which she endeavored to throw herself. It was with great difficulty that she was prevented from accomplishing her design. She remained insane during the rest of her life, which he adds, "was fortunately not long protracted." Such cases illustrating the frequency and intensity of the suicidal and homicidal propensity abound in every work on mental disease and are found in every asylum. But, on the other hand, there are undoubtedly many cases of suicide in which the hypothesis of insanity is untenable. Cato stabbed himself rather than live under the despotic reign of Caesar; Themistocles poisoned himself rather than lead the Persians against his countrymen; Zeno, when ninety-eight, hung himself because he had put his finger out of joint; and Hannibal and Mithridates poisoned themselves to escape being taken prisoners. When we search Scripture we find that Saul, rather than fall into the hands of the Philistines, commanded his armor-bearer to hold his sword that he might plunge upon it; Samson, for the sake of being revenged upon his enemies, pulled down the house in which they were reveling and "died with them"; and Judas Iscariot, after selling the Saviour for thirty pieces of silver, was overcome by remorse "and went and hanged himself." The examples quoted from ancient history show that the deed was the result of Stoic philosophy, and those from the Bible show motives sufficient for the act, and in all must we discard the theory of insanity.

To come down to our own times, we may take, for example, the case of Benjamin Hunter, the Camden murderer. For four or five days before his execution he made a practice of sitting over the prison register, with his legs covered by a blanket, and, under the pretense that they were cold, kept rubbing them with his hands, leading those who saw him to believe that he did so only for the purpose of increasing their warmth by restoring the circulation through them. Upon the night preceding the execution he managed to secrete a basin in which he placed his feet, and after cutting through the vessels with a piece of sharpened tin he commenced the process of rubbing, and was actually forcing out his life with every movement when his appearance attracted the attention of the keeper. His object had almost been gained, and, under the circumstances, can we say that it was an insane one? He was a proud man, who dreaded the disgrace of a public execution; he also possessed in a marked degree the desire to cheat the law of its deserts, which is a characteristic tendency of the criminal mind; in one constituted and situated as he was there were sufficient reasons to account for the attempt, and, instead of its being the act of a madman it was merely the effort of a determined will to accomplish a desired end. Cases innumerable might be cited, did space permit, where persons of undoubted sanity have committed suicide for the purpose of escaping suffering, punishment, or disgrace. In fact, a great many of the suicides of which we daily read, probably the majority, cannot be considered due to cerebral disease, but must be looked upon rather as the result of social laws, combined with false training and education.

"Is suicide ever justifiable?" is another mooted question, and many writers have answered it in the affirmative. Epictetus, Zeno, Pliny, Seneca, and Plutarch were its advocates. Hume, in his "Essay on Suicide," says: "It would be no crime for me to divert the Nile or Danube from its course if I could; where, then, is the crime of turning a few ounces of blood out of its natural channels?" Rousseau taught, "To seek one's own good and avoid one's own harm in that which hurts not another, is the law of Nature." Budgel believed that, "when life becomes uneasy to support, and is overwhelmed with clouds and sorrows, man has a natural right to deprive himself of it, as it is better not to live than to live in pain." Montesquieu, Montaigne, Dr. Donne, and others have advanced similar ideas; but it is needless to say that their arguments can find support only in the minds of those who believe that "death endeth all."

The tendency has always been to palliate the act, and the verdict, "committed suicide while laboring under temporary aberration of mind," has become a stereotyped phrase. This verdict was frequently rendered in earlier times for the purpose of preventing the property of the deceased from reverting to the crown, and it has been kept alive in more recent times by the desire, which is inherent in every human breast, to speak kindly of the dead. It is evident, however, that such a verdict should only be rendered when the actions of the deceased have been such as to point very strongly to insanity, or where the autopsy shows undoubted lesions of the brain. Under such conditions no other verdict would be just. But when one becomes "a deserter from the army of humanity," and resorts to suicide as a means of escape from the trials of life, the act is merely a confession of weakness, which, while it may awaken feelings of compassion, certainly does not call for palliation. There are conditions of life, I will admit, to which death might seem far preferable; but though our misfortunes may be such as to make us long for the grave, we must, to slightly change the noble words of Burke, "even in despair live on," remembering that—

"Our time is fixed, and all our days are numbered;
How long, how short, we know not; this we know,
Duty requires we calmly wait the summons,
Nor dare to stir till Heaven shall give permission."

Suicide and the Environment[2]

In the discussion of the increase of suicide in the United States, a great deal has been said in the consideration of the act as a crime, but little, comparatively, in reference to its causes or to those preventives which society has power to enforce. Dr. D. R. Dewey, who some years ago made a careful study of the question as it related to the New England States, declared that since the year 1860 suicide had increased in those States to the extent of thirty-five per cent. This percentage, with but slight variations, will probably apply to all other States of the Union where there is great industrial and commercial activity.

Suicide is so violent a reversal of that strongest instinct of Nature—the instinct of self-preservation—that its causes and preventives will always be the subject of deep and careful investigation. If it is on the increase, there must be causes for its increase, and these causes being ascertained, it is then our duty to

---

[2] By Robert N. Reeves

devise means for its prevention. Insanity, heredity, financial reverses, and domestic complications may be direct incentives to suicide, but back of them all is the real cause— the growth of a nervous, disordered temperament in the American people. The steady habits of our colonial ancestors no longer satisfy us, and, as a consequence, those amusements, those ventures and schemes which excite the mind and nervous system to the highest degree are becoming more and more prominent. This, no doubt, is the fundamental cause of all suicide. But it is only with the direct incentive that society is capable of dealing, and these direct causes are so numerous and varied that it is almost impossible to classify them with any degree of accuracy. The individual may be impelled to self-destruction by circumstances, by an innate craving or instinct, by an uncontrollable impulse, by the unhealthy reasoning of a disordered intellect, and by many other influences. Suicides may therefore be divided into two great classes—those in which reason is called upon to decide between life and death, and those which are due to impulse or insanity.

In the former class the self-destroyer has, after reasoning upon his condition, come to the conclusion that death is the most acceptable of impending evils. In this class may be placed all those suicides due to sickness, financial embarrassment, ungratified ambition, the desire to escape justice, and causes of a like nature.

Among the second class, or those self-murders which are the direct or indirect outcome of insanity, may be included all cases of persons who are impelled to destroy their lives when insane, of those who commit the act on some trivial cause or provocation or from imitation, of those who while sane give way to sudden impulse, and of those who, after a longer or shorter struggle, succumb at their own hands to a growing impulse. Civilization, drunkenness, imitation, and hereditary propensities are accountable for much of the self-destruction prevalent; and so, to a greater or less extent, are age, sex, the state of health, and daily occupations of the victim.

Attempts have been made to prove that climate has an effect upon the rate of suicide, but these attempts have never done more than show that the temperate regions have the highest ratio. This, of course, is not due to the climate, but to the more complicated civilization, the greater physical and mental wear, and the more extensive interference with natural laws met with in the temperate regions. While it is true that climate exerts but little influence over the rate of suicide, the seasons, on the contrary, do strongly affect it. The popular belief is that suicide is more frequent during the months of winter and spring. This, however, is incorrect. Cold, wet, damp weather does not, as so many people suppose, promote despondency and suicide. Strange as it may seem, at that period of the year when the sufferings of the poor and the sick are least, when employment is most readily obtained, when the pleasure of living should be at its highest, suicide is most frequent. May, June, and July, the months of song and sunshine in all countries, give the greatest number of self-murders. For this there is no satisfactory explanation, unless we accept that of the medical fraternity, which is that during the period of early summer the organism is working at a higher tension, every function of mind and body is more active than at any other period of the year, and consequently there is greater liability to sudden physical and mental collapse.

The sad fact that suicide and education increase at an equal rate is now generally admitted. Civilization does not free humanity from grief, disgrace, and disappointment; but wherever civilization is highest the struggle for existence is fiercest, life is most artificial, and there the most failures of the human race are met with. There was a time in Roman history when suicide was almost epidemic. It was when the great republic had reached its acme of civilization—when poetry, art, and eloquence were triumphant. It is probable that the proportion of suicides due to mental derangements is increasing, but how rapidly can never be exactly determined. Morselli says that about one third of all suicides may be attributed to insanity.

Many people, however, anxious to stamp the act with reprobation, declare that every suicide is insane. This is wrong. While those who bring about their self-destruction may have acted wrongly or unwisely, we have not the right to declare them all insane. It is true that many persons brood over their troubles until everything loses proportion, their minds become unbalanced, and in such a state they kill themselves. In such cases the act may be correctly attributed to insanity. But what are we to say of those who are to all appearance rational and yet are the victims of sudden or growing impulses? Such people are not voluntary agents, and yet they cannot be called insane. They are abnormal. There is a fatal defect in their organization which is incompatible with their survival under natural conditions. This defect may give rise to sudden impulses or may cause a growing gradual propensity which terminate in the final tragedy. Instantaneous impulses are often brought about by the slightest circumstances. Thus, gazing steadily at the wheels of an approaching train or looking down from some great height may produce a delirium, a distention of the blood-vessels of the brain, that instantly paralyzes the will of the victim.

In the consideration of those propensities which are of gradual growth we are confronted with an extremely difficult problem. We know that a great many of those who ultimately destroy themselves fight for years against the impulse. How are we to account in such cases for the persistence of the tendency toward suicide, which seems to be a part of their nature, a part which draws them instinctively to death just as the normal creature is drawn to a desire to live? For such cases heredity may be in a great measure responsible. It is clear that hereditary influences may reveal their force in the suicidal impulses as in many other of the problems of life.

Whole families have been known to kill themselves. There are a great many human beings who by nature are predisposed to self-destruction, and only wait through life for a calamity sufficiently great to prompt them to the act. They are victims of their own faulty organizations.

Individual temperament may have a great deal to do with the question of suicide. In America the population is largely composed of the various European races, and although these are living under the same conditions, each nationality retains its own peculiar rate of suicide. Drink and crime are responsible for a large proportion of the daily self-murders.

Drunkenness, the most active agent of degeneration known, is directly responsible for those which occur during a period of nervous depression following a debauch. Among the criminal classes suicide is quite common, but it is among the petty and not the grave offenders that it occurs. Poverty and disease are also strong incentives to self-destruction. Suicide is often regulated by the price of bread. Life has few pleasures for the homeless and friendless. Death to them is often a welcome friend, a happy relief from walking the streets hungry.

How many suicides are directly attributable to disease cannot be stated with exactness, but it may be said, nevertheless, that at the present time, with our advanced skill in surgery and medicine, suicide from disease is undoubtedly on the decrease. Of all suicides there are none to be pitied more than those who kill themselves to escape the racking pain of an incurable illness. For the victim of this sort there is no hope. Another class of suicides, which closely resemble those caused by disease, includes those due to infirmity. Often persons smitten with blindness, or who have met with some terrible accident, in a fit of discouragement kill themselves. Those blind or deformed from birth, however, seldom resort to suicide. Not knowing the pleasure of sight or limb, they go through life contented.

The theory that we hold more strongly to life as we approach its natural conclusion is contradicted by statistics, which everywhere show that the last half of life exhibits a great increase in the rate of suicide. And here it may be pointed out that as to the age of greatest frequency, suicide and crime are diametrically opposed. While suicide attains its highest rate after the prime of life is past, crime, on the contrary, reaches its highest point between the ages of twenty and thirty years. We remark, further, the alarming increase in late years of what is called child-suicide. It is here that education strongly asserts itself as a true and exciting factor, for it has been shown that in those countries where what we are pleased to call education is rigorously forced upon children, there child-suicide is most frequent. And for this system of forced education there is no excuse. It is terrible in its consequences. To increase the strain to just below the collapsing point is not to educate. It only serves to fill the world with nervous, neurotic, morbid beings.

Another cause of the increase of child-suicide is the fear of physical punishment. Instances of children destroying themselves because of punishment or the fear of threatened punishment are constantly recorded in the public prints. Repeated cruel punishments will often extinguish, even in the healthy child, the love of life so characteristic of youth. What, then, are we to expect of poor, devitalized children subjected to the cruelties of barbaric parents?

At the present day man is much more prone to suicide than woman. This is true of man in regard to epilepsy, crime, and other marked signs of degeneration. But it has been observed that as woman approaches man in her mode of life she also becomes more familiar with those abnormal conditions which have previously been peculiar to man. The comparative immunity of woman from self-destruction in the past has depended greatly upon the relatively less harassing part she has taken in the struggle for life. Today it is different. Now woman occupies the fields of art, literature, finance, and even politics, and, as she goes deeper into these vocations, she must expect to suffer the consequences. Already it is noticeable that feminine suicide is not now entirely due to the sentimental causes of disappointed love, desertion, and jealousy, but to those trials of a more material order such as have led men to the act of self-destruction.

Imitation far exceeds any other of what are called "trivial causes" of suicide, and asserts itself more in woman than in man. It is much more common than is supposed. When self-destruction becomes epidemic, as it sometimes does, its prevalence very largely depends upon imitation. It is said that many years ago the wail of Thomas Hood over The One More Unfortunate brought many a sentimental person to a watery grave in the Thames. And in our own day the vivid representation of suicide upon the stage under conditions appealing forcibly to the imagination has been known to be followed by the self-imposed death of persons whose conditions resembled closely those of the suicide in the drama.

The daily papers are largely responsible for this class of suicides. It can scarcely be doubted that the general diffusion of newspaper reports familiarizes too much the minds of the people with suicide and crime. A single paragraph, a chance expression, a cause given which resembles that of the circumstances surrounding the reader, seizes the imagination, and in a morbid excitement the desire to repeat the act is born. Newspaper reports further promote suicide by inflaming the passion for the notoriety which will be conferred upon the perpetrator through their accounts of the act.

Has city life any influence over the proportion of suicides? This question must be answered in the affirmative. Where the population is dense and the laws of health are neglected, where dirt is common and vice flourishes, where the poor are concentrated, and where fortunes are made and lost in a day, will always be found the highest rate of suicide. It is in the poorer districts of our large cities that suicide is most frequent. In these districts the deprivations of light and air, the poverty, the diseased conditions about them, render the poor moody, morbid, and despondent, and raise in their minds a feeling that life is not desirable.

What can society do to prevent suicide among the poor? The obvious method would be to render their conditions more enjoyable by giving them ampler provisions for pleasure and recreation, making their surroundings more cleanly and agreeable, and by faithfully executing thorough, and most effective sanitation. Proper sanitary and hygienic measures have a wonderful effect in renewing the vitality of our people. They are powerful agents for improving morality.

There probably never will be a time when suicide will be unknown in the world, but there are many preventives that are of value to-day. Religion has in the past been a powerful preventive. But this fear dies out as religion becomes broader. The fear of future punishment on account of self-imposed death is not now the preventive of suicide that it was fifty or a hundred years ago. The moral influences of family life naturally have a tendency to decrease suicide. Thus it has been found that in a million of husbands without children there were four hundred and seventy suicides, and in the same number with children there were but two hundred and five. Of a million wives without children one hundred and fifty-seven committed suicide, as against forty-five with children; widowers without children, one thousand and four; with children, five hundred and twenty-six; widows without children, two hundred and thirty-eight; with children, but one hundred and four. These figures are eloquent pleaders in favor of family ties as conservators of life. They prove distinctly that man must love in order to live.

Laws prescribing punishment for suicide are solecisms. If we wish to prevent suicide we must change conditions for the better, not for the worse. Suicide is beyond the reach of the criminal code. Its prophylactic must be founded, not upon a statute, but upon a wise and judicious management, medical, moral, and philanthropical, of those unfortunate enough to attempt their lives. It would be far better and more humane to sweep away all legislation upon the subject so far as it relates to the individual, and even take for granted that every person is insane who attempts suicide, than to punish their attempts by imprisonment. If the victim is insane, efforts should be made to restore reason; and if failure is met with, a sanitarium should be provided. Those who are sane should be reasoned with, calmed, and assisted.

Our hearts should be filled with tender compassion for those whose lives have been such as to become valueless to them. We should pity them. In the gentlest language possible we should condone and not condemn their act; for it is only with a spirit of sympathy and not of vindictiveness that we can hope to study with profit the causes and preventives of suicide.

Suicide in Large Cities[3]

The increased importance attached to the study of the relations of mind and body (the impetus to such study we have to thank Mr. Maudsley for) enables us to pursue our examination of certain psychical states to greater advantage than in former years. The investigation of suicide is now made much more clear as regards both the motive, behavior, and characteristics of the individual who takes his own life, and by the antecedents of his previous health, and other physical influences.

The object of this paper is to discuss the prevalence of this crime in large cities, its causes both moral and physical, and certain sanitary conditions which affect them. My observations have been made for the most part in New York, the largest city of the continent, and, as the most cosmopolitan, it offers an interesting field for research. I have made comparisons between the statistics of London

---

[3] By Allan McLane Hamilton

and Paris, and, although it is impossible to obtain the most recent records of these two cities, I think a few hints may be gained that will be of value in preventing its increase. Statistics do not give us definite information upon the questions of heredity, cerebral injuries, neuroses, or other valuable aid in drawing conclusions, so that many important links are left out of the chain.

In all large cities the number of suicides is governed, to a great extent, by the habits, tastes, and moral culture of the people, and, back of this, by the national characteristics. For example, the French, notorious for their indifference to life, their general volatility, frequent political troubles, and exaggerated morbid sentimentality, are celebrated for the propensity to end life by their own hands.

Paris has been, and always will be, celebrated for the prevalence of this crime. The late Forbes Winslow, in his "*Anatomy of Suicide*," called particular attention to this national failing of the French. They pursue it as an agreeable mode of getting relief from their troubles, and, from the statesman, who blows his brains out to escape political disgrace, to the *grisette* of former days, who shut herself up with her little pan of charcoal, to seek oblivion from her ruin, the crime is a general one, Montesquieu, on the other hand, asserted that the English are notably a suicidal race, and that London, with its fogs and cheerlessness, is more of a city for suicides than Paris. Forbes Winslow denied this, and demonstrated that fogs had no influence whatever upon suicides; or, at least, that there were fewer suicides in foggy months than in more pleasant ones. Our own statistics substantiate this, as will be shown further on, and the months of April, May, June, July, and August, really the most pleasant of the year as regard sunshine, are those in which more people kill themselves.

The gravity and stolidity of the English people would rather show in their favor as regards this crime. In the year 1810 the number of suicides in London amounted to 188. Comparison with French statistics of the same year proved that five times as many Parisians as Londoners took this means for ending their days. French statistics show the excessive mortality from this cause. In the year 1806, 60 suicides were reported in Rouen, an extremely small city; in 1793, 1,300 in Versailles. Paris, from 1827 to 1830, furnished 6,900 suicides, an average of nearly 1.8 per year. In recent years, we have better statistical returns to work upon.

In the year 1858 the population of London was 2,720,607, and the number of suicides 283. The youngest of these was ten years, and the oldest eighty-five. In Paris, in 1853, the population was 1,053,262. There were 463 suicides, an immense number in excess of London several years later. In Turin, from 1855 to 1859, there were 108 suicides, making an average of 21 a year. In Rome, in 1871, there were only 15 suicides, showing that self-murder is very uncommon among the Italians. In the city of New York, between the years 1866 and 1872, there were 678 suicides, being an increase of 100 in the last year over the first; 511 males, 167 females. For the three years, 1870, 1871, and 1872, there were 359 suicides, 132 being Germans, a very large percentage. As regards matrimonial condition during these years, I find there were 17 married persons, 118 single, 43 widows and widowers, and 27 whose condition was not stated; 275 were males and

84 were females; the age of the oldest was eighty-six, and that of the youngest ten.

The cause for the suicide of the latter was remarkable. She was detected in a theft of fifty cents, by her mother, and, to seek escape from her shame, took Paris-green. The months in which suicide was most prevalent were those of summer. In August, 1870, there were 15 suicides, while in December only 7. In June, the following year, there were 14, and July of 1872 shows 20, and December only 4.

In regard to occupation, clerks commit suicide the most frequently, about 34 in 1870, 1871, and 1872, and but 10 laborers in the same time. The percentage of laborers abroad is greater than any other. The mode of suicide most often employed in the city of New York is that of poisoning—212 out of nearly 600 persons have died from some form of poisoning. The preference seems to be for arsenic; usually its commonest form—Paris-green. In 1872, of 50 poisoning cases, 22 took Paris-green; the others chose either opium, carbolic acid, or other irritants. In 1871, 14 took Paris-green. Nearly all of the suicides chose violent and painful poisons, there being but few exceptions. One individual ended his days by hydrate of chloral; the other, a druggist, with prussic acid. Three took chloroform. Shooting ended the lives of 147 persons; 135 hung themselves. In only one or two instances was any ingenuity shown in the suicides: one of these individuals first shot himself, and then jumped out of the window; the other threw himself in front of an advancing locomotive. In London, hanging seems to have been the method most in vogue, for, in the year 1858, 56 persons perished in this way.

A. Brierre de Boismont, in his "Recherches Médico-Légale sur Suicide," Paris, 1859, collected 4,595 cases, carbonic-acid gas and drowning being the favorite modes for self-murder with men, and strangulation with women. Of 463 suicides occurring in the year 1853, 92 men perished by carbonic-acid gas, 93 by drowning, and 131 women died by strangulation. The more ancient statistics show that voluntary starvation was a common form of suicide in the beginning of this century. The motive for suicide in the reported cases was extremely difficult to discover. Of the 463 cases in Paris in 1853, insanity produced the suicide of 53 men, 37 women; drunkenness, 48 men, 14 women; misery and grief, 20 men, 8 women; disappointed love, 28 men, 20 women; shame, 18 men, 9 women; domestic trouble, 18 men, 15 women; weariness of life, 20 men, 7 women; disease, 27 men, 19 women; fear of the law, 16 men, 2 women; ill-luck, 23 men, 14 women; trouble with parents, 5 men, 5 women; loss of situation, 8 men; loss of parents, 1 woman. By this table, it will be seen that insanity causes the largest number of suicides, both of men and women; drunkenness comes next, and disease third.

In regard to the form of suicide with fire-arms, Boismont shows, by a carefully-arranged table, that the greatest number shoot themselves in the mouth, seventy-five per cent, choosing this means.

Out of 368 cases, 234 shot themselves in the mouth, 71 in the abdomen and thorax, 26 in the temple, and but 1 in the ear, thus showing a knowledge of the vital parts of the body. In illustration of the coolness and resolution of these suicides, he found that 85 left wills. The chirography of letters and various communications written before death was steady and natural, not betraying any signs of weakness, trembling, or irresolution on the part of the writers. Parisian statistics prove that of 3,518 cases, 2,094 occurred in the daytime, 766 in the evening, and 658 at night, proving that daylight is most agreeable for this kind of work. The ages at which suicide seems to be most often resorted to are between forty and fifty among the men, and forty-five and fifty-five among the women.

The greatest number of suicides in the city of New York, as I have said, are by poison, and this mode of self-destruction being the favorite one, we are naturally led to inquire why it should be so. When we take into consideration the looseness of our present laws regarding the sale of poisonous drugs, and the comparative ease by which suicides can procure the agents for their destruction, we have very little cause for wonderment. The number of cases of accidental death which have occurred through the criminal carelessness of certain druggists, who deal the most deadly drugs to persons unknown to them, is worthy of serious comment. There appears to be no difficulty for the would-be suicide to buy just what poison he desires. A large proportion of the inhabitants of great cities are confirmed in certain pernicious habits. Among them are opium-eating and chloroform-taking, which they pursue to what extent they choose, as these articles are always to be had.

It is needless to say that the opium-habit, like alcoholism, frequently leads to self-destruction.

In this country, upon several occasions, certain individuals have taken their own lives after insuring them, that the policy might be paid to the family of the suicide. This is an example of a very interesting psychical condition. Alcohol and its secondary effects have swelled the number of suicides, and the victims who have died by their own hands have been equally of the higher and the lower classes in this country. I think a great increase in the returns of mortality of this especial variety of suicide would be observed if the reporting physicians would conscientiously state the cause of death. The shame attached to the procedure, particularly among people of position, has prompted the return to be made of "meningitis," "cerebral congestion," or other diseases. Within the last two years, I can call to my mind the suicide of six people of high social position, caused by drink. This vice is perhaps not entirely characteristic of large towns, but the facility for indulgence of the habit, and the numerous ways of drinking in private, are more perfect in the cities.

In smaller places, there is a certain amount of contact with one's fellows, which makes him the cynosure of all eyes, should he indulge too freely. As I have before said, the busy life men lead in the metropolis, and the necessity for brain-stimulus, accelerate the *facilis descensus*. The disgrace of men in high position, impending ruin and other facts, will often prompt suicide as a mode of relief.

A form of suicide which figures largely in American statistics is, jumping from an elevation. This may be chosen by the individual as an effectual method, if he hesitates to select one, or may be the result of a momentary state of delirium produced by the surroundings. This latter is a common form in some European cities that contain high churches, monuments, or towers. I have myself experienced a morbid desire of this character, after an ascent of the Mountain Corcovado, in the harbor of Rio de

Janeiro. When looking over a steep precipice upon this bay, two thousand or more feet below, I felt a strange restlessness and distention of the blood-vessels, with an irresistible desire to leap out into the clear air. This disappeared when I looked upon some object nearby. A medical friend relates a case in his own experience. He went with an acquaintance up into a very high, unfinished public building. There was no evidence of insanity in his acquaintance. When my friend's back was turned, his companion jumped far out into the air, and fell mangled to the sidewalk. In France this form of suicide is a very common one, 45 individuals in the year 1820 having precipitated themselves from heights. In the year 1852, 16 men and 19 women chose this means of self-murder. So prevalent were those suicides, that the authorities refused admission to the Column Vendôme. As I have before said, this method is not an unusual one. In New York, between the years 1866 and 1872, there were 21 victims.

Dr. C. P. Russell, of New York, has informed me of a friend who is to such an extent the subject of the impulse to throw himself from heights, that he will never sleep upon the third or fourth floor of any dwelling.

The impulse to commit suicide with sharp-cutting instruments has been more common in the European cities than those of this country, and, in the majority of instances, suicide by these weapons has been resorted to by insane subjects.

A most important study in connection with this subject is the influence of the mode of life of the poorer classes. I allude more particularly to the tenement-house system—to the colonization of many thousand people in a limited space, much too small for them. They are brought together so, that every vice becomes, to a great degree, contagious. Bad examples are followed by the younger generation, and it is much easier for a seed of sin to take root here than one of virtue. Families of several nationalities are closely packed together in front and rear houses. Ground and labor are so expensive, in the larger cities particularly, that this mode of living is unavoidable.

Despite the earnest efforts of an efficient health board in the city of New York, many radical defects exist, and ventilation, light, and drainage, are defective in the extreme. Diseases of the nervous system, principally of the trophic character, exist to a great extent, as results of imperfect lighting and ventilating.

In the five years preceding 1872 the deaths from nervous diseases in New York averaged 3,155.8, and for the years 1871 and 1872 were over 6,000, an unusually large proportion, the number of deaths from all causes being 59,623. The vices attending the colonization of the working-class (a great many do not work) are contagious, the moral contact of the vicious with the pure is certain to occur, the ruin of young girls, and depression of tone, are powerful inducers of suicide.

The American people partake of the characteristics of their transatlantic brethren. They are impulsive, energetic, enterprising, emotional, liable to excessive mental depression or exaltation. We have all the different bloods of Europe in our veins. We lead, however, an individual life of our own, a life as original and striking as other startling peculiarities of our country. We live too fast; we make and lose fortunes in a day; we acquire professional educations in a few years which take ordinary individuals as many more to get the rudiments of in Europe. It is anything but *festina lente* here. The seeds of every national soil are sown, and take root before we can employ measures to suppress them. Everything that can excite the emotions, make tense the mental faculties, and suddenly relax them, is among us. Speculations and stupendous schemes, which in older countries take several heads instead of one to mature, crush down the nervous system of men who work themselves to death, hardly taking time to eat, meanwhile living upon stimulants to enable them to stand the strain.

There is another class—I allude to the poor. The newspaper accounts of the miserable suicide in his upper attic tell this story every day. These subjects are chiefly foreigners, deluded to this country by unfounded expectations of fortunes to be made.

Only a few days ago I read in one of the daily papers that it was not an uncommon occurrence for immigrants to ask of the officials at Castle Garden, in perfect good faith, positions as insurance officers, bank officers, and other unattainable positions.

Many thousand Italians were sent here by rascally agents in their own country several years ago. They were promised work by these individuals, but on their arrival found none. They reached New York in mid-winter, and many of them found their way into the workshops and almshouses. Misery and suffering were prevalent. Among immigrants, particularly the Germans, there is a great disposition to suicide, and physical suffering doubtless awakens any hereditary tendency that may lie dormant. A great percentage remain at the seaport, looking for work. New York is particularly affected in this way. Immigrants come here, probably in most instances from occupations much more steady and remunerative in comparison to any found here; trades-people, skilled workmen, and mechanics, often commit suicide, who find it difficult to obtain employment, and finally hunger and disappointment drive them to this step.

The prevalence of strikes, and trades-unions, with their dangerous restrictions and foolish oaths of allegiance, are fruitful causes of suicide. Men are afraid to work in opposition to the threats of their fellow trades-unionists, and, as poverty stares them in the face and they become desperate, they commit suicide.

A necessary attendant upon increase in population is immorality, engendered by vice attendant upon civilization. The more depraved forms of theatrical amusement found at the low theatre halls, two or three of which now exist in New York, wipe out all of the original purity from the nature of the weak-minded spectators. The low songs at some of these places, abounding in *double entendres* and suggestive gestures, inflame the dormant instincts of lust in the minds of the deeply-interested audience.

Prostitution is a very easy way leading to suicide. The attendant vices of this class very soon destroy the mind. Opium-eating, inebriety, and snuff-chewing, are habits which nearly all prostitutes follow after a time. The classification of these causes of suicide and their victims is very incomplete, and prostitution is placed on the records in only one instance in 1871, 1872, and 1873, as the calling of the individual.

The prevalence of seduction in large cities is perhaps greater among the lower classes—the workers in factories and shops. Indeed, the chance for this crime among the many thousand young girls and men who are herded together indiscriminately in the large tobacco, hoop-skirt, paper-box, and other factories of great cities, is often made use of. Suicide follows ruin, though not in as many cases as it would in France. I do not doubt but that the large rivers, upon which most American cities are built, give up a great many bodies of unfortunates who end their moral ruin by suicide. In fact, the number of cases reported as "found drowned" may be assumed in general to be suicidal.

In our own cities, as I have before shown, clerks seem to be the class that most often take their own lives. This seems reasonable when we consider the peculiar careers of a great many of them—the temptations of vice, the struggles for situation and support, and the pitfalls of a large city.

How shall we prevent the increase of this crime which advances at the rate of 300 per cent, in seven years? What sanitary measures can be taken to defeat its moral and physical causes?

It is a stupendous undertaking. To reduce its statistics would require an attack upon our whole social system.

I have pointed out the rapidity of our way of living, the excessive and unnatural strain upon the brains of business and professional men. To diminish this would be an almost impossible task. I can only suggest a diminution of working hours, the necessity for regular meals and habits, and means to prevent large cities from being over-stocked by the agricultural classes, who imagine themselves in these days particularly fitted for business and professional pursuits. We should abolish immoral entertainments, advertising quacks, so-called anatomical museums, and obscene and sensational literature, as far as possible.

Legislation should strictly regulate the sale of poisonous drugs, and the police should enforce the laws. Friends and relatives of excitable and nervous persons should be alive to the necessity of keeping from their reach razors, cutting instruments, and poisons. They should also endeavor, as far as possible, to prevent the formation of the opium-habit, self-administration of chloroform, and alcoholic indulgence.

Careful watch should be kept on all persons who go up into high public buildings, church-spires, and other eminences. Physicians should employ caution lest their patients should habitually indulge in some narcotic drug originally prescribed. The boards of health of the different cities cannot be over-zealous in suggesting means for the improvement of the dwellings of the poor. Air, light, and ventilation, should be provided, if possible, for these are absolutely necessary for nervous development and healthy cerebration. I have always considered the system of small dwellings, that has succeeded so well in Philadelphia and other cities, an inestimable boon to the working-classes. A healthier moral and physical tone is engendered, both by elevating the self-reliance of heads of families, and the abolition of moral contamination so prevalent in tenement-house life.

The establishment of bureaus and other agencies for procuring work for immigrants, freeing the cities from the surplus of these people, would prevent much desperation, misery, and self-destruction.

Suicide and the Weather[4]

Much has been written and rewritten on the subject of suicide. It has long been a favorite topic with the student of social statistics, and has been scientifically treated from the standpoint of race, of nationality, of social condition, of occupation and of climate. Whole volumes have been devoted to the problem and magazine articles almost without number. It is not, however, my intention in this paper even to summarize the conclusions arrived at in all this mass of literature, but to discuss a phase of the subject which cannot have escaped the reader of the daily paper, and has long proved an enigma to the special student of the problem of self-destruction—that is, the daily fluctuation in the occurrence of suicide. Why is it that upon picking up our daily paper one morning we see the heading 'Epidemic of Suicide', and find the details of six or eight or even a dozen successful or unsuccessful attempts recorded for the previous day—a number greater than for

---

[4] By Pr Edwin Grant Dexter

the whole week preceding? Yet such is often the case—so often, in fact, as not infrequently to have been the subject of editorial comment, with vague queries as to the cause of such a wave of emotional depression and consequent self-destruction.

The answers to this query have been many and varied, among the most frequent of which has been chance. Mimicry and suggestion have been proposed, and without doubt have their place in the solution of the problem of the periodical fluctuation of the suicide curve, but still cannot account for all its peculiarities. The weather has also been suggested as the cause of the fluctuation referred to, and it is to the following out of this promising clew that this paper is confined.

From *a priori* grounds it would seem to be a good one, for of all the environmental conditions, those of the weather are the only ones which vary for all the individuals in a given locality simultaneously. A and B and C all have troubles peculiarly their own, the climax of which could not be expected to occur upon the same day; but when the east wind blows and the sky is leaden A, B and C all feel the influence, whatever it may be, and an empirical study of large numbers of A's and B's and C's, noting their behavior under such conditions, would seem to be the surest method of discovering just what the influence is.

That weather states have a mental effect has long been recognized. Literature is full of allusions to the fact, and not a few of the world's great thinkers have left on record their own emotional flights and depressions under different meteorological conditions. But most of us need to take no other word for the fact than our own. In all the vigor of perfect health such influence may hardly be recognized, but when the vital powers are depleted by the exhausting effects of a long nervous or physical strain, then this phase of the cosmical environment is sure to make itself felt. Then come the days when everything goes wrong. The groundwork of forgotten quarrels is remembered, uneasy questions arise with regard to the future; one gets tired of life. And how much of all this can be attributed to an east wind or a leaden sky—in other words, to weather effects? In order to answer this question we must de- fine our use of the term 'weather effects.' From the standpoint of our present study we should include within the category of weather effects any marked inequality in the occurrence of suicide which may be found to bear a fixed relation to the fluctuations of what we call weather. We conclude that a fixed relation between a given weather state and an unusual prevalence of suicide is causal and not accidental. This is based upon an inductive study of large numbers of data, and is as valid as such studies can well be.

The problem, then, consists in discovering these fixed relations. In order to do this with exactness, the meteorologist's analysis of weather must be taken. To him a given weather state is a complex and not a simple phenomenon. He reads its temperature, its barometer, its humidity, its wind velocity, its sunshine or shade, and its precipitation, and it is only to the synthesis of these conditions that he applies the term weather. For the purpose of our present study it is not enough to say that the weather is fine, or disagreeable, or muggy, for those terms mean one thing to one person and something very different to another, so it has been necessary to make use of a definite meteorological nomenclature which is recognized the world over. The study is in no sense an attempt to account for suicide, but for the irregularity of its occurrence. Man always has sought and perhaps always will seek self-destruction as the relief for sorrow, fancied or real, and the basal reason for this is not to be found in the weather. We would not argue that the weather drives people to suicide save in very exceptional cases, but, on the strength of what follows, that under some weather states other things are peculiarly liable to drive people to the act. In other words, that some meteorological conditions so affect the mental state, so influence the emotional balance, that ordinarily endurable things become unendurable, and life seems no longer worth the living.

This problem, which seems to show a causal nexus between the weather and the mental state of the suicide, is a comparison of the occurrence of suicide under different meteorological conditions, with the normal prevalence of those conditions, noting the excess or deficiency. The data were collected for New York City and the city of Denver, Col., and although the climatic conditions of the two cities are very different, it is in no sense a comparative study for them. In fact, so few data (two hundred and sixty suicides) were procurable for the western town that but little weight is given to conclusions based upon them, compared with the much greater number for New York City, and the study of the former is only incidentally mentioned.

The method of procedure was as follows: In order to procure the proper data of suicide for the city of New York the records of the coroner for five years were carefully gone over (some 28,000 separate death certificates), disclosing the particulars of 1,962 suicides, and the exact number (varying from to 9) tabulated for each of the 1,826 days of those years. Next the police records for the same five years were studied, and the number of unsuccessful attempts for each day noted. This record is quite complete, since in the eyes of the law one attempting suicide is a criminal, and must be so branded on the books. From these two sources were obtained the exact number of persons who for each day of the period covered were of suicidal intent, unless some unsuccessful attempt escaped the surveillance of the police. In the present article neither age, sex, nationality, nor occupation is considered; simply the fact that someone wished to die by his own hand—for the five years, 2,946 in all for the city of New York.

When the data of suicide had thus been tabulated, the meteorological basis for the study was obtained from the records of the United States Weather Bureau. At the New York station (Denver for the Denver study) were copied the mean temperature, barometer and humidity, the total movement of the wind, the character of the day and the precipitation for each of the 1,826 days of the period considered, and placed opposite the already tabulated number of suicides. Then, by a somewhat laborious process of tabulation, the exact percentage of days which were recorded at the Weather Bureau under each of the seventy-seven definite meteorological conditions represented by the accompanying figures was computed. That is, the exact percentage characterized as 'clear,' as 'partly cloudy,' or 'cloudy,' as having some or no precipitation (without considering the amount), as having had a mean temperature between zero and five degrees F., between five and ten degrees, and so on for each one of the designated groups for temperature, barometer, humidity and wind. Now, it may be readily seen that these percentages represent the normal or expected occurrence of suicide for each meteorological group if the weather had no effect. For instance, if thirty per cent, of the days are found to be characterized as 'clear,' we should expect that same percentage of suicides for 'clear' days plus or minus the percentage due to probable error from accidental causes (which with the number of data used would be very small) if the character of the day had no influence on *their occurrence.* If forty per cent, did actually occur under such conditions, we should be forced to conclude that fair days were prolific of suicide, as indeed they seem to be. This principle was applied to each of the meteorological groups, and the figures show graphically the results.

For each, the general meteorological condition is indicated at the top; the definite group readings are given in small figures upon the heavy vertical lines which represent the occurrence of suicide for the group. Expectancy for each group is represented by the vertical distance A—B and excess or deficiency graphically shown in percentages of this, which may be read by means of the scale at the left.

The method of tabulation, by means of which the actual occurrence of suicide for each meteorological group, was determined was similar to that for expectancy, and needs no further explanation.

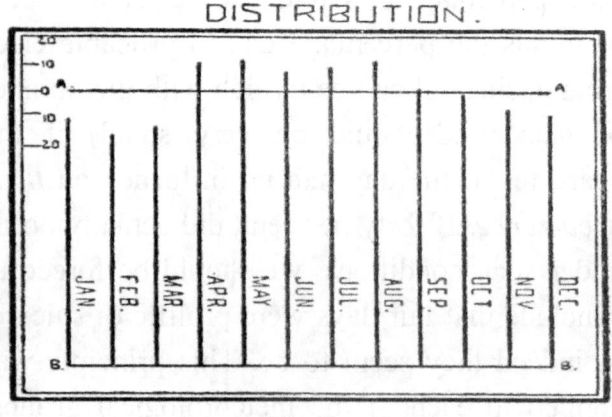

Fig. 1.

MONTHLY DISTRIBUTION.—Fig. 1 indicates very wide variation in the number of suicides occurring in the different months of the year—

generally speaking, the heated months showing excesses and the cold ones deficiencies when compared with the normal. May and August show the greatest numbers, with the least for February, in spite of the fact that the shortness of the last-named month is taken into consideration.

It may be seen, by an inspection of the figure, that the increase in number for each month from February to August, and the decrease for the other months of the year, would give an almost perfectly regular *crescendo-diminuendo* to the occurrence curve were it not for the fact that April and May are raised out of their position by unusual excesses. Why April, which in its general weather characteristics is Elysian compared with its immediate predecessor, should show one-fourth more suicides, and May, which by common acclaim is one of the most delightful of the calendar, should present a number surpassed only by sweltering August, it is not easy to see. Yet such is the case for the five years covered' by this study, and similar conditions have been demonstrated by other students of the subject. Morselli, in his exhaustive treatise for the

European nations, finds that for thirty-two separate studies made by him the maximum numbers were in June eighteen times and in May eight times. In explanation of the fact he says, "Suicide is not influenced so much by the extreme heat of the advanced summer season as by the early spring and summer, which seize upon the organism not yet acclimatized and still under the influence of the cold season." There is little doubt that the end of winter brings with it a depleted condition of vitality, both nervous and physical; yet I am inclined to think that the fact cannot wholly account for the great increase in the later spring months. In the conclusion of this paper the condition is again alluded to, and at this point I would simply call attention to the fact that the increase comes with the season of the year when rejuvenating Nature is in her brightest mood.

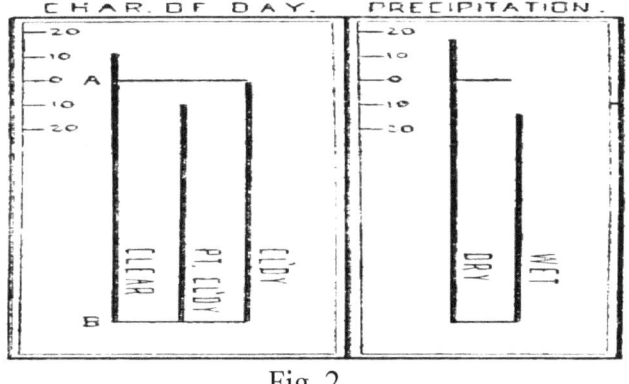

Fig. 2.

CHARACTER OF THE DAY AND
PRECIPITATION. — The terms 'clear' 'partly
cloudy' and 'cloudy,' as used by the Weather
Bureau's characterization of weather states,
have a definite and technical meaning. The first
is used to designate days on which the sun is
obscured for three-tenths or less of the hours
from sunrise to sunset; the second from
fourtenths to seven-tenths of that period; and
the third eight-tenths or more. (See Fig. 2.)

Under precipitation I have considered
separately days which were absolutely free
from rainfall or snowfall, and those on which
there was either, without considering the
amount.

The figure referred to discloses some unexpected facts—namely, that the clear, dry days show the greatest number of suicides, and the wet, partly cloudy days—the gloomiest of all weather—the least, and with differences too great to be attributed to accident or chance; in fact, thirty-one per cent, more on dry than on wet days, and twenty-one per cent, more on clear days than partly cloudy. As will be seen, on cloudy days the occurrence was about normal. What does this mean? Must fiction resign her right to ring in gloomy weather and blinding storms as a partial excuse for ending an existence made more unendurable by these? If such be the case, it is well that Dickens and Lytton and Poe are gone, for they would be robbed of a large number of their tragic climaxes. England has long been characterized as 'gloomy Britain,' and Montesquieu has called it the 'classic land of suicide, ' stating that the 'excessive number of suicides for that country is due to its gloomy weather.' Statistics have shown, however, that the number is not excessive there, being less per million inhabitants than for any other important European nation. An interesting paper, appearing in the British magazine Once a Week (vol. xix.) over no signature (though the writer was evidently not a Scotchman), has a bearing upon the subject. It says:

"The idea that the prevalence of suicide in this country (England) is due to our bad weather is precisely one of those hasty and illogical inferences which are characteristic of the Gallic mind. The constant gloom of bad weather ought to acquaint us so thoroughly with moods of depression that suicide would never occur to us. Look at Scotland, for instance, where suicides are rare. Why are they rare? Simply because a succession of Scotch Sundays has so accustomed the people to prolonged despondency that any sudden misfortune cannot sink their spirits any further. One has only to spend a dozen Sundays in Glasgow or Edinburgh to become inoculated against suicide. So far from London fogs driving people to jump off Waterloo Bridge, they ought to train the mind to bear any calamity. A man who has taught himself to eat prodigious quantities of opium feels scarcely any effect from other forms of intoxication. We can educate our mental susceptibilities as we can our muscles, and the more we educate them the more they are able to bear."

There are many truths beneath the jocular vein of this quotation, and the writer expressed more facts than perhaps he knew.

Certainly a comparison of suicides for Denver and New York City supports his theory, for in the former city, where cloudy and partly cloudy days are less than one-third as frequent as in the latter, we find suicide excessive during the gloomy weather. Yet the conditions there, both social and climatic, are so unusual as to give this fact little weight in a comprehensive study of suicides, and we must maintain that Vilemais's dictum that 'nine-tenths of the suicides occur in rainy or cloudy weather' is utterly unfounded upon fact, at least for the conditions covered by this study.

TEMPERATURE.—Fig. 3 seems. to show plainly two things:

(1) That the greatest excesses of suicide are found at the two extremes of the temperature scale, when the conditions entailed the maximum of actual misery, and

(2) that the next greatest excesses occur during the pleasantest conditions of temperature.

I would here, however, call attention to the fact that for all the figures the readings at the extremes of the conditions are based upon fewer data than those nearer the middle, hence are more liable to accidental error. For example, although the temperature group zero to five degrees shows an excess of two hundred and ten per cent., the condition occurred but twice in the five years studied, and the whole number of suicides was but eight, while the excess of fifteen per cent, for the group sixty-five to seventy degrees is based upon two hundred and sixty-eight. For this reason the value of the readings at the extremes of all the figures, except Fig. 1 and the upper limit of Fig. 5, at which point there were data enough to give validity to the findings, is lessened when compared with other points in the curves.

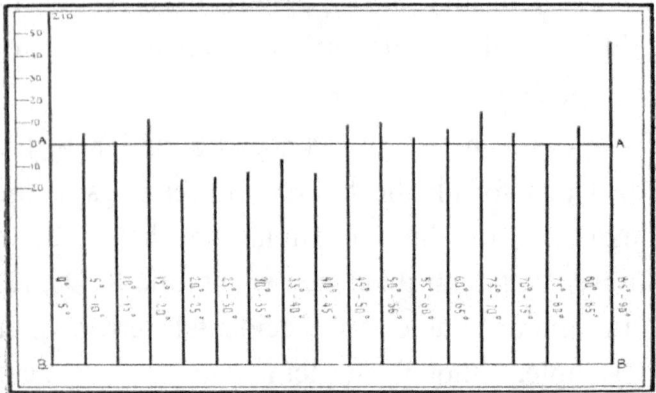

Fig. 3.

Taking this fact into consideration, the greatest numerical excesses in suicide occur in the temperature group from forty-five to seventy degrees. This places them within the category of most agreeable temperatures, for within those limits are found the monthly means of April, May, June, September and October. The deficiencies of suicide occur in the groups from twenty to forty-five degrees, conditions which are not generally considered most agreeable and within which are found the monthly means for the colder months of the year.

These results, however, are corroborative of the findings for the study of monthly occurrence which show deficiencies for those months. The excesses for extreme conditions of heat and cold are perhaps only what might be expected. In the thickly populated tenements of the city great heat becomes so oppressive as hardly to be endured, and at the other extreme of temperature, when the mercury of the thermometer is only in the bulb, both personal misery and a feeling of sympathy for a dependent family might prompt one to self-destruction as the last resource.

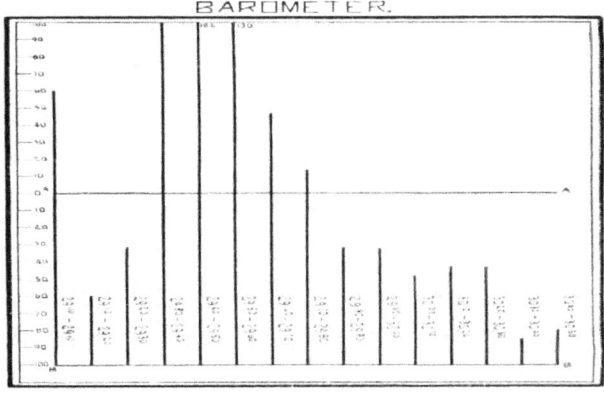

Fig. 4.

This curve does not differ materially from that of the Assault and Battery, except that in the latter it is shown that for the highest temperature ever experienced those misdemeanors, as recorded by the police, show deficiencies. For them the numbers increase regularly up to a temperature of eighty-five degrees, but above that point they fall off very rapidly. This fact, however, is not hard to account for, since a considerable amount of energy is required to be objectionably out of order, and at such conditions of heat this seems hardly available.

BAROMETER. — Considering the liability that accidental conditions affect the validity of our curves at their extremes, the results shown in Fig. 4 prove conclusively that low conditions of pressure are accompanied by excesses in suicides, with corresponding deficiencies for the re- verse barometrical readings. We cannot, however, suppose that it is the actual density of the atmosphere which produces this marked effect. A difference of pressure as great as that between the two extremes for New York City would be experienced in going to the

Adirondacks, and five times as great in a trip to Colorado, without producing tendencies to personal annihilation, so we must look for our explanation elsewhere. It is probably to be found in the relation which exists between atmospheric pressure and some other weather states—possibly storms. The peculiar mental and physiological conditions which prevail for a considerable period just preceding violent storms or marked changes of weather have long been recognized, and it may be that in them we have the solution. Persons afflicted with gout or rheumatism, or even corns, can 'feel' the approach of such meteorological conditions, and certain mental peculiarities are probably just as prevalent. Many weather proverbs are based upon the unusual activities of members of the animal kingdom at such times, and as a storm is often preceded by a low condition of the barometer, we have perhaps an explanation of their cause. More work, however, must be done to demonstrate this as a scientific fact.

HUMIDITY.—The results of the study of suicide for this condition (Fig. 5) are in themselves conclusive, but directly opposite to those found in similar studies made for Assault and Battery, Deportment in the Public Schools and the New York City Penitentiary, and the behavior of the insane. For suicide the excesses are for high humidities; for the others mentioned they were for low.

The showing for suicides seems to be what would be naturally expected if we were to theorize on the matter, as those unendurable 'sticky' days, when one feels it his prerogative to be 'out of sorts,' are usually of high humidity. There are some interesting conclusions to be drawn here by a comparison of this curve with that for precipitation. The latter showed deficiencies of suicide for rainy days, while this gives an excess for humid ones. Now, all rainy days are humid, but not all humid days are rainy, and our logical conclusion must be that the excesses shown by the present figure must have been for the humid variety, yet without precipitation. Such precisely is the 'sticky' weather mentioned, and its effect must have been deadly to produce such results.

In accounting for the unusual number of assaults and misdemeanors in the public schools for low humidities, as discussed in the paper cited, the electrical potential of the atmosphere for such meteorological conditions was considered the cause. It is a fact conceded by scientists that at every point upon the earth's surface there are lines of electrical force extending off into space, and that the potential is roughly in a reverse ratio to the humidity prevailing at a given time. This electrical condition for regions of universally low humidity, as the altitudes of our western plateaus, is very marked and productive of no slight effects. These seem to be a mental and even physical exhilaration, productive of energy which in the long-run generally proves to be in excess of the normal healthy possibilities. The result is for those regions a tendency to overwork, especially mentally, with a resulting state of collapse. Although these conditions are not so marked for the higher humidities of the sea level, they nevertheless exist to a degree, and without doubt in New York City there is less individual surplus energy when the humidity is relatively high than when relatively low. This would lead us to infer that, from the showing of this condition, suicide was excessive when energy was low.

This relation of occurrence to available energy is reversed for certain of the figures, but other conditions enter in which are discussed in the conclusion of this paper.

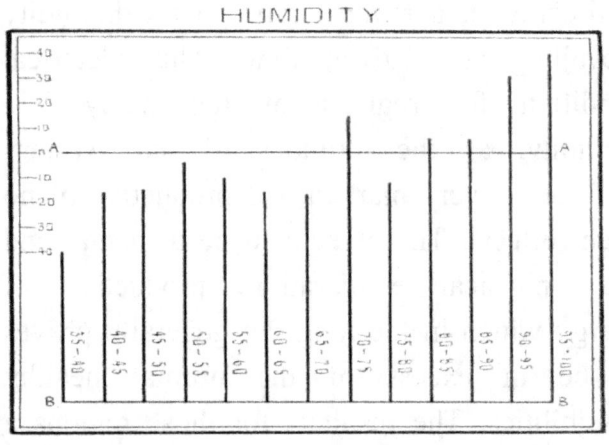

Fig. 5.

WIND. — But little need be said upon the effect of this factor as shown by Fig. 6. The regularity of the increase of suicide with increase in movement of the wind is too marked to allow any other theory than that of a causal nexus. This effect seems to be much greater upon the suicide than upon any of the offenders mentioned in the study cited. It is, however, shown to be as great or even greater for all classes of crime in the Colorado climate, where wind is an important factor in the production of high electrical states. The other study, however, showed very slight wind effects for New York City, and their comparison with this would seem to prove that the mental states of the suicide and of the street brawler are very differently influenced by it.

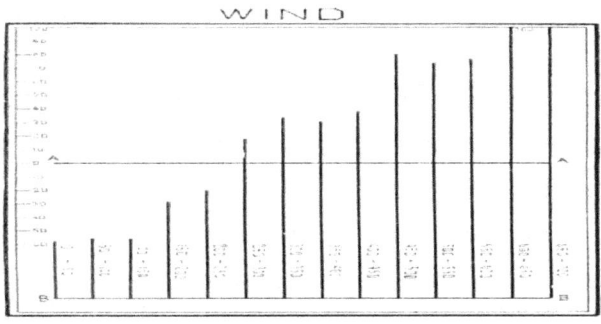

Fig. 6.

It is difficult, in conclusion, to summarize the results of this study in such a manner as to be of much value or to bring forward theories which are certain of any long tenure of life. The whole method of the study is too new and untried, and the number of data inadequate. The bare facts revealed in the preceding paragraphs must prove of much more value than any hypothesis drawn from them at this stage of the investigation. Still, there are a few generalizations which seem worth noting, especially as they are based in part upon findings which are entirely contradictory to popular opinion with regard to the time chosen by the suicide for the final act.

The first is that suicide is excessive under those conditions of weather which are generally considered most exhilarating and delightful— that is, the later spring months and upon clear, dry days. Reference to Figs. 1 and 2 proves this conclusively for the number of data and the locality studied. It was also noted that there were the greatest numerical excesses for the most agreeable temperatures. Barometrical conditions can hardly be referred to the categories agreeable and disagreeable, but for humidity and wind the relation will hardly hold, since we have the greatest excesses during high humidities and great wind velocities, both of which are unpleasant. Yet these facts would not invalidate our first statement, for neither high winds nor great humidities bring a scowl upon the face of Nature that can be compared with that of a wet, drizzling day. In fact, a day may be bright, and be both windy and humid. Yet these latter conditions have effects peculiarly their own, as shown conclusively by the study of deportment already cited. They are, for wind, the production of a neurotic condition in which self-control is in a marked degree lessened, and for high humidities the production of a minimum of vital energy. The former is shown especially in the study of the school children, and the latter of the death rate. These facts make it possible for us to amend our statement that suicides are excessive during the most noticeably delightful conditions, by adding: coupled with especially devitalizing ones.

But this does not in any way account for the seemingly anomalous effect of bright weather. To me the only plausible hypothesis is that of contrast. Investigation has seemed to prove that very few suicides are committed on the 'spur of the moment.' The act is generally pre-meditated, and its consummation deferred, sometimes again and again. We can hardly doubt, either, that it is dreaded, and the hope entertained, even to the end, that it may not need to be. During the winter months that hope must be centred on the belief that when Nature smiles with the spring sunshine all will be well; on the gloomy day, when the morrow comes with its exhilarating brightness, the present cloud of un- happiness will be gone. The love of life is still strong, and the grave cannot be sought while there is still hope for better things.

But spring comes with all its excess of life, and the morrow with its brightness, but do not bring to the poor unfortunate, unable to re- act to these forces as of yore, the hoped-for relief. He thinks of other springs when the bluebirds sang happier songs, and of other sunshine which had set his blood tingling. The drowning man had waited long for the straw; it came and he clutched it, but it sank beneath his weight.

Genius and Suicide[5]

Winslow in his Anatomy of Suicide, says, "A person who accustoms himself to live in a world created by his own fancy, who surrounds himself with flimsy idealities, will, in the course of time, cease to sympathize with the gross realities of life," and anyone who will take the trouble to read the biographies of men of genius will see that this statement is borne out to a remarkable degree. Probably the most striking example of this doctrine, as well as the most pathetic instance of suicide in the annals of literature, is found in the records of Chatterton's short life. From the beginning shadows hovered over him. He was the posthumous child of a poor widow, whose dead husband had been a rough, drunken fellow, and a singer and subchanter in the cathedral choir of Bristol. The mother supported herself by dressmaking in one of the back streets of the old town, and the boy was only able to gain the rudiments of an education in a charity school.

[5] By Charles W. Pilgrim

His biographer tells us that he was of a peculiar temper, sullen and silent, and given to sudden fits of weeping or violent rage. When only ten years of age he began to write verses, and although he was too shy and diffident to make a confidant of any one, his secret soon became known among the little blue-coats of Colston's Charity School. His uncle, Richard Phillips, was the sexton of the church of St. Mary Redcliffe, in Bristol, one of the most beautiful specimens of parochial church architecture in all England, and many of this strange boy's days were passed studying the inscriptions on the altar tombs and in poring over the forgotten parchment deeds which had lain for years unheeded in the oaken chests in the old muniment-room above the porch. So much of his time was spent in solitude, and he seemed to have so few of the characteristics of children, that many regarded him as weak in intellect. But even then he was thirsting for fame, and while only a child was wont to say that a man might do anything he chose. It was the accidental discovery of the old parchment deeds in the parish church that led this child of genius to perpetrate the Rowley forgeries, and to claim that these products of his own imagination had lain in the old chest for more than three centuries. Failing to obtain the patronage of Sir Horace Walpole, he determined to seek his fortune in London, and in order to obtain his release from Lambert, an attorney into whose employ he had been bound, he sat down on Easter eve, April 17, 1770, and penned his Last Will and Testament, in which he intimated his intention of committing suicide. Among his satirical bequests he leaves his "humility" to the Rev. Mr. Camplin, his "religion" to Dean Barton, and his "spirit and disinterestedness" to Bristol. This strange document had the desired effect, and Lambert canceled his indentures. So, with a light heart, a lighter purse, and a bundle of valuable manuscript under his arm, he set out, at the age of seventeen, to gain fortune and fame as a man of letters in the great metropolis. His afterlife is well known. Nothing but disaster followed. He lacked the simplest necessities of life, but even when starving wrote cheerful words and sent small gifts to the mother and sister left behind. Failure met him at every hand, and by degrees he sank lower and lower into the depths of despair, until finally, with his last penny, he purchased sufficient arsenic to end his unhappy life. He was found on his cot of straw with torn manuscript all about him. Thus ended the brief, strange life of the "fatemarked babe who perished in his pride."

Another example of Winslow's doctrine is Hugh Miller, the self-taught genius, who was born at Cromarty, in the north of Scotland, on the 10th of October, 1802. Like Chatterton, he had little patience with the schools. He would play truant in order to enjoy a book in freedom on the hill or by the sea, and his old schoolmaster feared that he would become a dunce. Curious to state, when it became necessary for him to decide upon a trade, he chose that of stone-mason so that he might be unemployed in the winter frosts, and thus have opportunity to read and write.

For fifteen years he worked in the quarry during the pleasant days of summer, and spent the hours of winter prosecuting the object of his ambition—the writing of good English. His clear, choice diction caused the Edinburgh Review to ask, "Where could this man have acquired his style?" little thinking that the greater part of his life had been spent in the quarry and hewing-shed.

His work attracted so much attention that in 1840 he was called to the editorial chair of The Witness, a semi-weekly paper published in Edinburgh for the purpose of securing spiritual independence. Unremitting labor resulted, and the night following the completion of his greatest work, The Testimony of the Rocks, he yielded to the strain to which his overworked brain had been subjected and sent a bullet through his heart.

Another similar case is that of Robert Tannahill, a Paisley weaver, who was one of the most popular successors of Burns in song-writing. He was born in 1774, apprenticed to his father's trade when twelve years of age, and composed his songs as his shuttle went to and fro. He apparently had a single love affair, which occasioned the composition of the popular song, "Jessie, the Flower of Dunblane." He was shy, sensitive, and awkward, and therefore uncomfortable except in the presence of his humble friends. His monotonous existence was broken only by occasional trips to Glasgow, and the one memorable day in all his life was when James Hogg, the Ettrick Shepherd, paid him a visit. The meeting was prolonged into the night, and the parting was painful and pathetic. Tannahill, grasping the hand of his poet-brother, said, while tears suffused his eyes: "Farewell! We shall never meet again." His words were prophetic, for shortly afterward his body was found stark and stiff in a pool near his house.

To come down to more recent times, we have but to recall the melancholy end of Richard Realf, an English peasant, born in Framfield, Sussex County, June 14, 1834. I cannot better give the story of his life than by quoting freely from a letter written to Rossiter Johnson in 1875, who was at work upon a short biography of the poet for the Little Classic Series. In this letter he says: "I never received any education in my boyhood, except for a year or two at the little village school. We were a large family and very poor, and I went to work in the fields at a very tender age." At fifteen, or thereabouts, he states that he began to write verse, "lisping in numbers, for the numbers came." When sixteen he went to visit his sister, who was a servant in the family of a physician at Brighton, and the wife of the doctor, who was a lady of literary tastes, manifested an interest in him and made him her amanuensis. A physician, who lectured on phrenology, shortly afterward became a guest of his benefactress, and learning of the young poet's ventures made use of some of them in one of his lectures to illustrate the organ of ideality. Among the listeners was Lady Byron. She with Rogers, Mrs. Jameson, and Lady Jane Pell, determined upon publishing a collection of his verses, and did so in 1852, under the title of Guesses at the Beautiful. He soon realized that he was in danger of being spoiled by condescending patronage and praise, and therefore wrote to Lady Byron, who was then at her country residence in Surrey, begging her to get him away from surroundings which might make him forget the honest peasant parentage from which he sprang. She at once made arrangements for him to go down to Leicestershire to her nephew, Mr. Noel, manager of one of her estates, where he would have opportunity to study the science of agriculture as well as to prosecute his literary purposes. Like all men of poetic temperament, he had the fatal faculty of falling in love, and an attachment soon sprang up between himself and the eldest daughter of Mr. Noel. Realizing that there was a gulf between them which could never be bridged, he determined to come to America. Reaching New York in 1854, he began to explore the slums for the purpose of writing sketches, but instead became a sort of Five Points missionary. He kept at this work for two years, and then in 1856 conducted a large number of Free State emigrants to Kansas. He became intimate with John Brown, was with him at Harper's Ferry, and narrowly escaped lynching. He enlisted in 1862 and served through the war with credit, rising by promotions to the rank of captain. The next step in his history has a local interest for us who live in the western part of New York, for in the autumn of 1867 we hear of him in Rochester writing a series of remarkable poems for the Rochester Union. It was there that Rossiter Johnson, who was then assistant editor of the Democrat and Chronicle, became interested in him, and it was also there that he contracted the unfortunate marriage which darkened his life and ultimately brought it to an end. Johnson, who has written fully of this episode, tries to excuse him by saying that the woman had nursed him through a critical illness, and that his gratitude made him believe that he could find peace and contentment where an ordinary man would have known that nothing but disappointment and unhappiness would follow. Realf himself said that he thought his mind was obscured at the time. After some years of misery he procured a divorce and remarried. Happiness seemed to be near again, but after two years, upon some technical grounds, the Superior Court reversed the decision of the lower court and declared his divorce illegal. Misfortunes then began to fall thick and fast. His second wife and children, for he had become the father of triplets, grew ill. Additional heavy drains were made upon his purse by a widowed sister and a paralytic brother, and to add to his cup of bitterness his first wife followed him to California and insisted upon claiming support. At last, bowed down and broken by misfortune, worry, and overwork, he ended with laudanum his eventful and unhappy life in the autumn of 1878. He made two attempts before success resulted, and between them composed the poem beginning "De mortuis nil nisi bonum," thus reminding us of Marcus Lucanus, "the eminent Roman poet of the silver age," who repeated lines from his poems descriptive of death as his lifeblood ebbed away.

If we were to look carefully into the histories of the lives of men of genius, we should find many names to add to the number already mentioned, and still more to swell the list of those who had attempted the deed without meeting with success.

Haydon, the celebrated historical painter and writer, overcome by debt, disappointment, and ingratitude, laid down the brush with which he was at work upon his last great effort, Alfred and the Trial by Jury, wrote with a steady hand "Stretch me no longer upon this rough world," and then with a pistol-shot put an end to his unhappy existence.

Richard Payne Knight, the poet, Greek scholar, and antiquary, was a victim of melancholia, and finally destroyed himself with poison.

Burton, the vivacious author of The Anatomy of Melancholy, who had the reputation of being able to raise laughter in any company, however "mute and mopish," was in reality constitutionally depressed, and it is believed that he was at last so overcome by his malady that he ended his life in a fit of melancholy.

Kleist, poet and dramatist, brooded over suicide, attempted it once unsuccessfully, and finally, by agreement with Henriette Vogel, who believed herself affected with an incurable disease, repaired to a small inn near Potsdam, where they ended their lives together.

Lessmann, the humorous writer, like Burton, put an end to himself in a fit of melancholy.

Sir Samuel Romilly, a man of brilliant genius, by whose efforts the criminal laws of England were remodeled—a man loved for his sweet nature and upright manliness—while overcome by grief at the death of his wife, with his own hand sought rest beyond.

Michael Angelo, after receiving a painful injury to his leg by falling from a scaffold while at work upon The Last Judgment, became so melancholy that he shut himself in his room, refused to see any one, and "resolved to let himself die." Fortunately, his intentions were frustrated by the celebrated physician Bacio Rontini, who learned by accident of his condition.

Vittoria Alfieri, of whom it has been said that every event in his life is either a factor of disease or a symptom of mental alienation, attempted suicide in Holland, while making one of his restless trips through Europe in search of change.

Kotzebue, who at last met a tragic death at the hand of an assassin, was at one time so melancholy that he meditated self-destruction. Happily, however, as he tells us, his habit of composition was so firmly fixed that he went on with his work and produced one of his finest dramas, Misanthropy and Repentance.

Cowper, as is well known, when bowed down by religious melancholy, made two unsuccessful attempts upon his life.

Chateaubriand, the brilliant representative of French literature, became so thoroughly discontented with himself and the world that he attempted to take his life.

Dupuytren, the distinguished anatomist and surgeon, whose kindly nature induced him to leave a large share of his fortune for the establishment of a benevolent institution for the relief of distressed medical men, contemplated suicide even when at the acme of his fame.

Cavour, "the regenerator of Italy," and one of the greatest of modern statesmen, twice attempted to kill himself.

Lincoln, as Herndon tells us in The True Story of a Great Life, was subject to fits of extreme melancholy. Nicolay also says that beneath his apparently cheerful and sunny nature there was an undercurrent of deep sadness. At one time, according to Herndon, his melancholy reached such proportions that his friends, "fearing a tragic termination, watched him closely day and night." At this time Lincoln himself wrote: "I am now the most miserable man living. To remain as I am is impossible. I must die, or be better, as it appears to me." While thus suffering he wrote and published a paper on suicide. But, to the glory of civilization, the shadows lifted, and he lived to place his name in perpetual honor by freeing the nation from "the incubus of slavery."

Lamartine, poet, statesman, and orator, when overcome by reverses which were as sudden as his successes had been, looked longingly toward the tomb.

George Sand declared that, whether it was that bile made her melancholy or that melancholy made her bilious, she had been frequently seized by a desire for eternal repose.

Goethe, who thought the suicide of the Emperor Otho worthy of praise, slept for several nights with a dagger under his pillow, trying to get up sufficient courage to imitate the act.

Comte, in a fit of depression, threw himself into the Seine; and there is abundant evidence that Shelley, whose unhappy life was clouded by the suicide of two women, himself contemplated the deed. Fanny Imlay's death by laudanum in the Swansea inn was followed in a few weeks by the recovery of Harriet Westerbrook's lifeless body from the Serpentine. The tragic death of Harriet was a frightful blow to Shelley, and there is no doubt that his character was altered by it. Thornton Hunt says, "I am well aware he had suffered sorely, and that he continued to be haunted by certain recollections which pursued him like an Orestes"; and Woodbury adds, "From that time a shadow fell upon him which never was removed." Whether it was the recollection of the watery grave of the woman he had wronged, or whether it was only the desire to rend the veil which hides the mysteries of the Great Beyond, it is certain that Shelley on more than one occasion contemplated self-destruction.

In Trelawney's interesting records of Shelley and Byron two striking instances are given. The first is a letter from Lerice, dated June 18, 1825, in which the poet writes: "You, of course, enter into society at Leghorn. Should you meet with, any scientific person capable of preparing prussic acid, or essential oil of bitter almonds, I should regard it as a great kindness if you could procure me a small quantity. It requires the greatest caution in preparation and ought to be highly concentrated; I would give any price for this medicine. You remember we talked of it the other night, and we both expressed a wish to possess it. My wish was serious, and sprang from the desire of avoiding needless suffering. . . . I need not tell you," he adds, "that I have no intention of suicide at present, but I confess it would be a comfort to me to hold in my possession that golden key to the chamber of perpetual rest." Notwithstanding the denial that he contemplated suicide, an incident which happened soon afterward, and which is related by Trelawney in the same interesting chapter, leaves no doubt that Shelley more than once felt the suicidal impulse to an almost irresistible degree. To make free use of Trelawney's graphic words: "On a calm, sultry evening, while Jane (the wife of Shelley's friend Williams) was sitting on the sands before the villa on the margin of the sea with her two infants watching for her husband, Shelley came from the house dragging his skiff. After launching her, he said to Jane: 'The sand and the air are hot; let us float on the cool, calm sea; there is room with careful stowage for us all in my barge.' She accepted the invitation, and, with the children, got into the boat. They soon drifted from the shore, and the poet, unconscious of her fears or of their danger, fell into a deep reverie, probably, as Trelawney suggests, reviewing all that he had gone through of suffering and wrong, with no present and no future. Jane spoke to him several times, but her remarks met with no response. "She saw death in his eyes." Suddenly he raised his head, his brow cleared, and his face brightened as with a bright thought, and he exclaimed joyfully, "Now let us together solve the great mystery." "With a woman's instinct Jane knew that her only chance was to distract his thoughts, and, suppressing her terror and assuming her usual cheerful voice, she answered promptly: "No, thank you, not now. I should like my dinner first, and so would the children." This gross material answer to his sublime proposition so shocked the poet that he was brought back to himself, and paddled his cockleshell boat into shallow water.

A deep melancholy pervades all of the poet's letters from Pisa and Leghorn, and it was at this time that he was engaged upon The Triumph of Life, which was left unfinished by his untimely end. The poem closes abruptly with these words: "Then what is life? I cried." A sentence of profound significance, as Mr. Symonds says, when we remember that the questioner was now about to seek its answer in the halls of death. "With all this evidence before us that death was not unwelcome when it came on that fatal Monday in the winds and waves, is it not fair to assume that had it not come as it did a record of suicide would have been added to one of the most interesting as well as one of the most melancholy histories in the annals of English song?

The examples mentioned have been taken at random, and I am well aware that an exhaustive search would have made this paper many times as long. My only aim has been to cite a few prominent examples in illustration of a subject which to my mind is one of fascinating interest, and to draw, if possible, some deductions from them.

Evidence is not lacking to warrant the assumption that genius is a special morbid condition, and the anthropological school of which Lombroso is the brilliant master is daily gaining converts. Although the doctrines which he advocates have recently received a remarkable impetus, they are not essentially new. Centuries ago Seneca taught that there was no great genius without a tincture of madness, and Cicero spoke of the *furor poeticus*. It is also more than a hundred years since Diderot exclaimed: "Oh, how close the insane and men of genius touch! They are

chained, or statues are raised to them."
Lamartine speaks of the mental disease called
genius; Pascal says that extreme mind is akin to
extreme madness; and everybody is familiar
with Dryden's couplet:

"Great wits are sure to madness near allied,
And thin partitions do their bounds divide."

This is not a pleasant theory I will admit,
but, as Lombroso says, does not the botanist
find the same thing; and "has not Nature caused
to grow from the same germs and on the same
clod of earth the nettle and the jasmine, the
aconite and the rose"?

But even though this view be not fully
accepted, if we take into consideration the fact
that the poet lives in an ideal world surrounded
by creatures of his own imagination, to whom
he attributes the most exaggerated sentiments, it
seems to me reasonable to believe that sooner
or later unhealthy introspection must be
awakened and followed, not infrequently, by
the development of morbid tendencies.

But, above all else, it is my belief that a lack
of proper training in the early years of life was
at the bottom of the unhappiness and mistakes

in nearly all the cases mentioned. In the lives of Chatterton, Miller, Tannahill, and Realf, the ones which we have the most closely analyzed, we find a similarity of conditions truly remarkable. Each was born to poverty of the direst kind, each had but little systematic training, and each drifted about upon the sea of knowledge until stranded upon its shoals. If these unhappy lives teach us anything, they certainly show the necessity of guiding with the utmost care the physical, the moral, and the intellectual course of the erratic child of genius. The precocious child especially should receive our most careful attention, for there is more than a grain of truth in the old adage that "genius at five is madness at fifteen." I am myself convinced that precocity is quite as often an indication of morbidity as it is of genius. In rare instances it fulfills its promises, but it only does so when the overactive and unequally developed brain receives proper nourishment and judicious exercise. If the early training be wrong, disappointment is sure to result, and "the huddled knowledge," as Disraeli says, "like corn neglected in a well stored granary, perishes in its own masses."

www.ingramcontent.com/pod-product-compliance
Lightning Source LLC
Chambersburg PA
CBHW060348190526
45169CB00002B/523